Frequently Asked Questions

all about
garlic

STEPHEN FULDER, PhD

AVERY PUBLISHING GROUP
Garden City Park • New York

The information contained in this book is based upon the research and personal and professional experiences of the author. They are not intended as a substitute for consulting with your physician or other health care provider. Any attempt to diagnose and treat an illness should be done under the direction of a health care professional.

The publisher does not advocate the use of any particular health care protocol, but believes the information in this book should be available to the public. The publisher and author are not responsible for any adverse effects or consequences resulting from the use of any of the suggestions, preparations, or procedures discussed in this book. Should the reader have any questions concerning the appropriateness of any procedure or preparation mentioned, the author and the publisher strongly suggest consulting a professional health care advisor.

ISBN: 0-89529-886-4

Printed in the United States of America

10   9   8   7   6   5   4   3

Contents

Introduction

Are you worried about your health? Are you anxious about your heart, or about the possibility of contracting cancer? If so, you are not alone, and your concerns are quite valid. Cancer and heart disease are today's major killers. If you are like most Americans, you are wondering how to beat these two deadly diseases and how to improve your health, without using medications that might have unpleasant or even risky side effects. Perhaps you've asked yourself if there is a safe, reliable, and cheap all-around preventive remedy that you could take every day, and that would help prevent some of these dangerous health problems.

There is such a remedy. And it may surprise you to discover that this remedy is available right at your local vegetable store. The remedy is called garlic. Believe it or not, garlic can bring about amazing improvements in your health, and can also help you prevent or combat serious illnesses, such as cancer and heart disease.

Garlic has become one of the most popular and talked about natural remedies of all time. Sales of garlic supplements in the United States have rocketed to several hundred million dollars per year. In Europe, where it is considered to be the number one remedy for the heart, around 5 million people take garlic daily. It is constantly in the media. Garlic has always been popular and for centuries was reputed to contain health benefits, but many doctors dismissed these notions as "old wives' tales." What's new is that its vital importance as a health aid is at last becoming recognized, even in the conventional medical world. Rigorous scientific research is convincing today's doctors to take garlic seriously. For example, the German Health Ministry has determined that garlic is a medicine for "preventing age-related deterioration of the circulation."

The research has confirmed that garlic is one of the best preventive remedies of all time. Garlic can lower cholesterol safely and easily. It can thin the blood and reduce blood pressure, making it a wonderful all-round remedy for the circulation. In addition, garlic can be used as a household standby for colds, catarrh, chest and throat problems, mouth infections, candida, and many other mild chronic infections. Garlic boosts the body's immunity and kills invading bacteria and fungi. It is excellent at cleaning the body by removing chemicals, waste, and toxins. It is also an excellent cancer preventive. Research has shown that garlic is the most helpful food in the prevention of cancer.

This book is a practical guide to using garlic as a daily remedy. It tells you what you can use garlic for, how it works, how much you should take, and for how long. The book explains how to incorporate garlic into a total wellness program, and what you can do if you have specific health problems, such as high blood cholesterol. *All About Garlic* mentions a few of the thousands of research studies confirming garlic's effectiveness.

Lastly, this book will address one of the most common concerns that people have when they hear about the wonderful and healing properties of garlic. No matter how interested people may be in improving their health, most don't want to become like the garlic-eating King Henry the Fourth of France, whose breath "could fell an ox at twenty paces." This book will teach you how to take garlic without the bothersome smell, and how to find your way through the maze of garlic products and supplements that clutter the shelves of supermarkets and health foods stores.

1.

The People's Medicine

Garlic is used both as a food and as a medicine. It grows nicely in all kinds of climates and is cheap and easily available. Because it can help with a wide range of common health problems, it is the number one household remedy for people all over the world. In this chapter, you will meet the garlic plant and learn about its many uses. For those with green fingers, there are instructions on growing garlic at home. We will briefly discuss the surprising fact that many spices can be safe and effective medicines, then we will focus on garlic and suggest when to use it as a food, and when to use it as a medicine. Finally, we will confirm that you can take garlic without any fear of side effects, and that even the smell can be avoided.

Q. What is so special about garlic? What will it do for my health?

A. Garlic has many different health-enhancing qualities. It addresses three major aspects of health: It is the key to a healthy heart, it is instrumental in cancer prevention, and it is a powerful way to treat infection.

Garlic is the foremost natural remedy to protect your heart and circulation. Since heart disease is today's leading cause of death, this simple herb could be a key to saving lives. It is a remarkable herb that prevents heart disease in several ways at once. Garlic lowers the levels of fat and cholesterol in the blood as effectively as many modern drugs now used for the purpose. Reduction of excess fat and cholesterol is one of the most important ways to prevent heart disease. Garlic, even in small amounts, thins the blood and helps to prevent clots inside the blood vessels. Since these clots can cause heart attacks and strokes, garlic may be able to reduce the risks of these health catastrophes. Garlic can also lower blood pressure. So we see that garlic addresses heart disease in several important ways that work together.

In addition, garlic makes us sweat and removes toxins from the body. It can stimulate the immune system and clean out cancer-causing chemicals. There is a great deal of research showing that there are substances in garlic that help prevent certain forms of cancer, especially those caused by toxins in the environment.

The other central use of garlic is in the prevention and treatment of infections. Garlic is safer than antibiotics. Extensive laboratory tests have demonstrated that garlic has a broader range of action than any modern antibiotic, even though it is somewhat milder and less potent. So you can use garlic to help treat nagging infections, including colds; coughs; bronchitis; sinusitis; laryngitis; infections of the stomach, such as gastroenteritis; infections of the skin, such as athlete's foot or ringworm; and infections of the urogenital areas, such as thrush or cystitis. It may be particularly effective against *Candida* yeast infections, a growing modern problem.

We see that garlic offers multilevel protection to an extent that no single modern drug is able to provide. And here's the best news of all: It is a food that millions of people eat daily without any ill effects. No wonder it has been praised for thousands of years as one of the main health aids known to mankind, a readily available and inexpensive preventive that should be in every household kitchen and medicine cabinet. No wonder that it is described in history as "The People's Medicine."

Q. Are we talking about the same garlic that I use in my cooking?

A. Yes. The garlic plant that is used as a medicine is the same one that is used throughout the world as an essential flavoring. It adds richness, taste, aroma, and nutrients to meat, fish, and vegetable dishes in Asian, Chinese, Middle Eastern, Mediterranean, European, and most other ethnic cooking.

Q. How can garlic be both a food and a medicine?

A. Foods can be medicines, and medicines can be foods. In fact, the popularity of garlic as a health supplement led to a cartoon in *The New York Times*. The cartoon showed a bemused consumer reading a "Prescription Only" sign posted over the vegetable aisle at the supermarket.

There really is a pharmacy on your kitchen shelf. Familiar examples include fiber for digestive problems, vegetables containing beta-carotene to prevent cancer, fish oil or olive oil to help prevent heart disease, cloves for pain, thyme for sore throat, cilantro or fenugreek seeds to adjust blood sugar, and artichoke for the liver.

Spices are on the borderline between food and medicine. It is perhaps hard to visualize those dry old powders in their bottles at the back of the kitchen shelves as being actual medicines. But most of them have definite therapeutic effect. Cloves, for example, will exercise an anesthetic effect on a sore tooth. Ginger can get rid of nausea. Many ordinary culinary herbs are actually medicinal foods. There is a huge traditional knowledge on how to use foods to prevent and treat disease. I experienced this first-hand during my two-year teaching visit to India. I was astonished to find that the village woman who cooked for us was designing the spice mixtures not just for taste, but for the season, the weather, and the health problems within the family.

Q. Why bother with spices if we have modern medicines to take when we're sick?

A. Culinary herbs such as garlic have some distinct advantages over modern drugs. In the first place, they are extremely safe. They are also inexpensive and readily available all over the world. Culinary herbs and spices can be effective in areas where modern drugs would be too strong and unnecessary. They can treat many mild common household health problems, from indigestion to headaches. Unlike most drugs, which treat diseases but don't prevent them, medicinal foods can be powerful preventive tools. Spices have some important nutritional benefits, providing extra vitamins and minerals that are absent from many modern medicines. Last but not least: Spices taste good. They are more palatable than capsules or tablets. They add zest and flavor to your foods and make eating much more enjoyable.

Q. Are the health benefits of garlic and other spices destroyed by cooking?

A. To some extent, but not entirely. The health benefits of garlic and other medicinal foods are partly destroyed by the high temperatures of cooking, as well as the length of time they're cooked. The longer the food is cooked, the smaller the quantity of medicinal ingredients that will be left at the end. Those ingredients not destroyed by the heat will be released into the air, which is why your neighbors might complain about (or enjoy) the spicy aromas that waft into their houses while you cook. The aromatic constituents that evaporate into the air during cooking are often valuable, health-enhancing ingredients.

So to get the full dosage and medicinal benefit from garlic and other spices, it may be necessary to take them separately from food. As a general rule, regard spices within food as having a mild preventive effect, and spices separate from food as having a stronger medicinal action. For example, a few seeds of fennel in your vegetable soup will have a gentle calming effect on your digestion, but fennel tea will be more effective in treating stomach gas. Similarly, garlic used in cooking will have a mildly positive effect on your circulation, but if you have a cholesterol problem, then you should take an appropriate dose of uncooked garlic. This is discussed more fully below.

Q. So what exactly is garlic?

A. Garlic is a close relative of onion, chives, and leeks. Botanically it is known as *Allium sativa*, and it belongs to the lily family. Like the onion, it has a solid round smooth stem and narrow, flat, spear-shaped leaves. The name garlic in fact comes from the Anglo Saxon *garleac*, meaning "spear-leek." It is a little larger than the onion, growing to about two feet tall. A cluster of purple-white flowers grows out from the top of the stem. The base of the stem is expanded into a fat bulb, which, when dried, is the garlic you find in the supermarket. This bulb or head of garlic contains from eight to fourteen cloves, each enclosed in a white papery sheath. Each clove weighs between one-tenth and two-tenths of an ounce.

Q. Is garlic easy to grow? Can I grow it myself at home?

A. Garlic is one of the easiest of all plants to grow. It can grow in almost any climate, from the tropics right up to the coldest parts of the United States. It is also not very fussy about the soil, and is not sensitive to most pests and diseases.

If you wish to grow garlic, plant the cloves about two inches deep with the tip pointed upwards. They should be a minimum of six inches apart. The planting time is late autumn, or early spring if the weather is particularly cold. The plant likes good but not very rich soil, which should not be too wet. Each clove will make a plant that will gradually develop a new bulb at the bottom. In July, pull up the plants, and hang them in bunches in a cool and dry place to gradually dry out. The dried plants will keep for a year or more. You can try braiding them as they do in France, and hanging the braids of garlic to decorate your kitchen.

Q. Are you sure that garlic is quite safe to take daily? Are there no side effects?

A. Garlic is absolutely safe. Some people occasionally experience heartburn, or some mild digestive discomfort. But this can happen only after eating fresh garlic, not garlic supplements, and it passes rapidly. Some people develop eczema from cutting and handling a lot of garlic. (This is often called "cook's hands.") Skin problems incurred through excessive handling of garlic can easily be remedied, and certainly have no relevance to the normal use of garlic as a supplement. There are no reports in the medical literature about negative side effects. Indeed, in some studies, volunteers have been given an entire head of garlic daily for as long three months without ill effects.

Of course, there is the smell, which is the main reason why some people turn their noses up at garlic. But medicines don't always taste or smell good, so an unpleasant odor can hardly be called a "side effect." And the smell can be dealt with, as we'll discuss later in this book.

2.

The Answer to Cholesterol

With heart disease at the top of the list of killers in today's United States, any help for this problem is important for all of us. In this chapter you will learn how garlic addresses heart disease. First we will discuss what heart disease is, and why it occurs. We will then focus on cholesterol, explaining what it is, and how it contributes to heart disease. You will learn how to incorporate garlic into a wellness program designed to prevent or treat heart disease: how effective garlic can be at reducing cholesterol, how much garlic you need to accomplish this amazing result, how long it takes to work, how garlic achieves this miracle, and whether you should take it if your cholesterol is not particularly high.

Q. I have heard of people getting heart attacks without even knowing they had any problem. What is heart disease, and what are its symptoms?

A. Heart disease is the result of a gradual deterioration in our circulation over many years. This deterioration takes place because our modern lifestyle includes many negative factors that affect the heart, such as unhealthy food, a sedentary lifestyle, and a great deal of stress. Also, since modern science has given us many ways to live longer, heart disease has many more years in which to show itself.

The cause of heart disease is a gradual and invisible blocking of the arteries. A blocked artery can be compared to a drain that slowly becomes obstructed by accumulating layers of solids. The blockage to the arteries may start with slight damage to the artery lining. The damaged area attracts small cell pieces called platelets. Platelets are a normal and healthy part of the blood, since they are crucial to the clotting process. If our bodies lacked the ability to manufacture blood clots, an injury might make us bleed to death. Under ordinary circumstances, platelets remain in the blood without becoming attached to the walls of the blood vessels, but once the platelets are attached, then sticky cholesterol globules, always present in the bloodstream, join the platelets. More and more cholesterol accumulates at the site and the result is a fatty deposit or plaque. In time, the deposits so swell the interior surfaces of the blood vessels that the passageway becomes partially blocked. The blockage is called a sclerosis, and the process of blockage is known as atherosclerosis. When severe, the fatty deposits precipitate the blood clotting mechanism, normally reserved for sealing up cuts. Clots (known as thromboses) form inside the blood vessels. The vessels that seem to be most at risk are those that bring the blood to the hardest working muscle in the whole body—the heart. A clot that stops up these vessels prevents blood from reaching the heart, causing chest pain, angina, or if more severe, a heart attack.

Q. What causes heart disease?

A. Several factors have been clearly identified as the main causes of heart disease. These are the ones you should watch for in your own life. If you find any of these factors to be relevant to you, then consult a doctor to assess whether your circulation or heart has already been damaged in some way. You should also address each of the risk factors to avoid any damage that might occur in the future.

These risk factors are a high proportion of animal fats and other saturated or hydrogenated fats in the diet, smoking, high blood pressure, high blood cholesterol, high blood sugar, insufficient exercise, obesity, and stress. Stress is sometimes difficult to recognize, but it plays a crucial role in heart disease. If you feel tense, anxious, pressured, or burnt out, or if you find yourself unable to relax, then you are suffering from stress.

There are secondary dietary factors to keep in mind as well. They include insufficient intake of vitamins and minerals, particularly the antioxidant vitamins C and E, magnesium, and B vitamins. People whose diet is imbalanced often lack these crucial nutrients.

Q. Is cholesterol ever good for the body?

A. Cholesterol has become almost a dirty word that people regard with dread because of its association with heart disease, but under ordinary circumstances, and within a normal range, cholesterol is an important component of good health. It is a fat that the body uses in the manufacture of a variety of important materials, particularly the male and female hormones.

Q. So if cholesterol is good for the body, how can it contribute to heart disease?

A. A normal amount of cholesterol in the blood is necessary for good health, but too much cholesterol definitely leads to heart disease. The excess cholesterol accumulates along the artery walls, leading to the growth of plaque, decreased blood flow, and eventually—if left untreated—complete blockage of the blood vessels.

Q. Is there any scientific evidence to show that high cholesterol contributes to heart disease?

A. An enormous number of scientific studies and statistics have supported the link between high cholesterol and heart disease. For example, animals fed a diet rich in cholesterol suffer from heart disease, while animals fed an ordinary diet do not. A fascinating study compared two different human populations: men living in East Finland and men living in Japan. The males of East Finland had the highest level of blood cholesterol in the world. They had an average of 265 mg of cholesterol to every 100 ml of blood. Japanese men, on the other hand, had an average of 160 mg of cholesterol to every 100 ml of blood. The heart attack level in East Finland was fourteen times greater than in Japan!

These findings have been confirmed again and again in scientific studies. A 10-percent reduction in cholesterol brings down the incidence of heart disease by 20 percent. In America, the average blood cholesterol level has gone down by 15 mg per milliliter of blood in the past thirty years. This reduction can be attributed to dietary changes and increased involvement in fitness-oriented activities. Heart attacks have been reduced by as much as a third during that time, and the average lifespan has increased by three years. These are impressive figures indeed, and they point to an indisputable connection between cholesterol levels and heart disease.

Q. While cholesterol levels have gotten lower in th U.S., has this been the case in other countries?

A. Sadly, the answer is no. The World Health Organization has looked at cholesterol levels worldwide and has stated that, for cardiac health, they should be at a maximum of 200 mg per 100 ml of blood. Unfortunately, two-thirds of the adult population of modern, post-industrial countries have cholesterol levels well above this figure, and suffer from a great deal of heart disease.

Q. How can that situation be remedied?

A. Some medical authorities have suggested that all such people take cholesterol-lowering drugs. This idea is absurd. It would make the majority of adults in developed countries feel like patients. It would create many undesirable side effects. The best way to combat high cholesterol and its negative consequences is to use safe, natural, and inexpensive means, such as a sensible exercise program and a low-cholesterol diet that includes culinary medicines, such as garlic.

Q. How do I find out what my cholesterol level is?

A. It is a wise precaution to go to your family doctor for a cholesterol test. Your doctor will take a little of your blood and send it to a laboratory for analysis. If your cholesterol is below 200 mg per 100 ml it is considered normal, or average for our society. A result of 200 to 270 mg per 100 ml is a gentle warning sign that you should take better care of your circulation. Above 270 mg per 100 ml is a danger signal. You should aggressively begin a cholesterol-lowering program, under the supervision of your health care professional.

Q. I have heard there is "good" cholesterol and "bad" cholesterol. What exactly are these?

A. Cholesterol does not simply float around in oily drops. It is packaged inside little bags of protein, which help it to dissolve in the blood. There are two main types of cholesterol/protein bags, called LDL (low-density lipoprotein) and HDL (high-density lipoprotein).

LDL is considered the "bad" form of cholesterol, since it is the one taken up by arteries to create fatty lumps. HDL, on the other hand, may actually provide a protection against heart attacks. It seems to act as a kind of housecleaner, collecting the cholesterol from the walls of the arteries and returning it to circulation. For these reasons, the HDL/LDL ratio is very often used as a measure of cardiovascular risk: the higher the ratio of HDL in the blood, the better the person's chances for avoiding heart disease.

Q. How can diet help to lower my LDL cholesterol?

A. Diet can make a very great difference to the level of good and bad cholesterol in our blood. A healthy diet can dramatically reduce the chance of a heart attack or stroke. In fact, a strict, well-chosen diet is the only way that is proven to be able to return the LDL level to what it was when we were born. It has been found that a pure vegan diet, with no dairy products, eggs, or meat, will achieve this result. Vegetarians usually have less LDL, together with more HDL, and, therefore, have a lower likelihood of cardiovascular problems.

Hundreds of studies have demonstrated that animal fats have the unfortunate result of increasing LDL cholesterol. This is now well accepted. But animal fats are not the only offenders. The total fat content of the diet contributes to the problem and should be decreased. In Japan, which has the lowest heart disease level of all developed countries, dietary fat makes up around 12 percent of the total food intake, while in the United States the percentage is three times as high.

A study compared 24,000 non-smoking vegetarians to the same number of non-smoking meat-eaters. The study demonstrated that the meat-eaters were three times more likely than the vegetarians to suffer a heart attack.

Fat is not the only dietary culprit in high cholesterol. Other dietary constituents are converted into fat by the body, in particular sugar and alcohol. Years of excessive alcohol or sugar consumption can keep the liver producing excess fat and sending it out into the circulation, adding to the LDL cholesterol.

Q. So a high-fat diet is not the only factor contributing to high cholesterol?

A. A diet high in fat is the most important factor, but by no means the only one. Keeping your diet low in fat is helpful, but there are other components to a healthy, balanced diet. A well-balanced diet should include essential vitamins and minerals, as well as plenty of fiber. Without these basic items, the liver is stimulated to manufacture too much cholesterol.

Lifestyle is almost as important as diet. Exercise burns up body fats, and a sedentary lifestyle causes those fats to build up. Stress is also a prime offender. The liver makes extra cholesterol if the body is under continuous stress. The extra cholesterol is needed to manufacture the hormones that the body requires to cope with the stress.

Certain illnesses or physical conditions also contribute to high cholesterol. Obesity, diabetes, and hereditary tendencies all play a role in determining cholesterol levels.

Q. What would I have to eat to maintain normal cholesterol levels?

A. Positive constituents of the diet include leafy vegetables, fruit, nuts, and seeds. All food fiber is helpful, especially the soluble fiber of fruit and vegetables. When the liver has generated too much cholesterol, it converts the cholesterol to bile and dumps it into the bloodstream. Food fiber ties up the excess cholesterol, making sure that it is passed out of the body through the intestines. Fish and fish oil are also kind to the circulation. They thin the blood, helping to reduce cholesterol and also to discourage the clotting process.

If you are like most Americans, you would be well-advised to cut your fat consumption in half. When you do eat fat, pay attention to the type of fat you consume. Saturated, or hard fats, including animal fats, margarines, butter, and palm oil, all contribute to atherosclerosis. The unsaturated vegetable oils, such as soy, sunflower seed, or safflower oils, are better for the circulation. Be aware that even these highly unsaturated vegetable oils should not be used excessively, as they can reduce the levels of the helpful HDL. The best oils for the heart are the monounsaturated oils, in particular olive oil. The heavy consumption of olive oil is one of the reasons that the level of heart disease is relatively low in the Mediterranean countries.

In addition, wholesome unprocessed foods are always healthier than refined and processed foods. For example, whole grains are better for our circulation than refined bleached flour. Many essential micronutrients, which can be costly if taken in supplement form, can be found easily and inexpensively in natural, unrefined foods. These include the antioxidants, such as vitamins C and E, as well as essential fatty acids, beta-carotene, zinc, copper, selenium, and magnesium.

Spices and herbs are wonderful additions to the diet, and contribute to the health benefits of genuine ethnic cuisine. After all, it is among them that we find garlic.

Q. Is garlic really an effective cholesterol-lowering remedy?

A. Garlic is unparalleled as a means to lower the cholesterol level. It is becoming accepted as a safe cholesterol-lowering remedy, even within the conventional medical community, and it has been the subject of a great deal of medical literature and clinical research. Around thirty clinical studies from research centers all over the world show that garlic, at a dose of only one to two cloves a day, will lower cholesterol by around 15 percent. This is enough to reduce the risk of a heart attack by 30 percent!

A study that was completed in 1988 in Germany looked at forty middle-aged people with high cholesterol levels. Their initial average was 295 mg per 100 ml. This is a dangerously high level. Most doctors would advise people whose blood contains such a high level of cholesterol to immediately start taking cholesterol-reducing medication. Half of the group took garlic products equivalent to one clove a day for three months. The other half were given a neutral, look-alike preparation. The cholesterol levels of those taking garlic dropped steadily over the three month period to an average of 233 mg per 100 ml, a decrease of more than 20 percent. Those taking the placebo pill did not show similar reduction in cholesterol and remained the same. None of the garlic-takers suffered any negative side effects. On the contrary, they felt more active and energetic by the end of the test period than they had been at the beginning.

A large study of high-cholesterol patients was carried out by Professor F. H. Mader and colleagues in Germany. The patients were divided into two groups.

Half of them took eight small garlic tablets (equivalent to less than a clove) per day, while the other half were given placebo pills. After sixteen weeks, the average cholesterol level of the garlic group was around 10-percent less than at the beginning of the study. Even more amazing, the higher the cholesterol level prior to the study, the greater the reduction by the end of the study. Interestingly, very few of the participants in the trial even noticed an odor from the tablets. A similar study by Dr. A. K. Jain and colleagues at Tulane University confirmed that garlic tablets were as effective as modern drugs for people with moderately raised blood cholesterol.

Q. Does garlic lower all types of cholesterol? Will it affect my HDL?

A. Garlic reduces LDL levels, while HDL is either unchanged or increased. This has been confirmed in many studies, with people as well as animals. For example, at the U.S. Department of Agriculture Research Laboratory in Wisconsin, researchers fed pigs a normal diet with additional garlic extract. Levels of LDL cholesterol fell by half, while the helpful HDL cholesterol increased by 20 percent. This is the same result that can be obtained by the most powerful modern cholesterol-lowering drugs, such as simvastatin or lovastatin. In a clinical study published in the medical journal *Atherosclerosis*, sixty-two patients with heart disease and sixty-two healthy individuals were given garlic. Over eight months, the healthy people reduced their LDL cholesterol by 15 percent, and their HDL increased by nearly as much. In the group with heart disease, the cholesterol fell by a massive 30 percent by the end of the study.

Q. Does garlic reduce cholesterol levels in everyone, even if they have normal levels of cholesterol?

A. The clinical research shows that everyone who takes garlic will experience some reduction in cholesterol. The extent of the reduction depends on how high the cholesterol is in the first place. Garlic can make a great difference in the cholesterol level of those with a genuine cholesterol problem. People with normal levels of cholesterol, on the other hand, may experience only a small reduction. This is illustrated by studies conducted in India. People whose cholesterol levels were normal, below 200 mg per 100 ml, had only minimal reduction, while those in the risk area—above 250 mg per 100 ml—reduced their cholesterol levels by as much as 25 percent.

Q. So should I take garlic if my cholesterol is normal?

A. If your cholesterol is genuinely low, you do not need to be concerned about it. The question is whether your cholesterol is actually as low as you think. In our Western society, "normal" is defined as below 200 mg per ml. Doctors are still debating whether this definition is really accurate. For example, the norm in Japan is lower than the norm in the United States, because most Westerners have elevated cholesterol levels. This makes the norm (or average) in Western countries higher than elsewhere in the world. This is a relative, not an absolute, measure. So even if you have a "normal" number, it may nevertheless be too high, and you may benefit from small, regular amounts of garlic. Besides, garlic has other helpful functions, such as cleaning the body of toxins, and lowering cancer risk.

Q. Does garlic work quickly? Will it reduce cholesterol if I take it along with a steak?

A. Garlic works immediately. If you eat a heavy meal with plenty of animal fat, your cholesterol level will increase within a short time. But if you eat garlic with your meal, it will help the body to dispose of the fat and cholesterol safely. This is why garlic is added to so many meat dishes—it is the traditional way of helping the body get rid of the waste. For example, Korean food is meat-based and is cooked with a great deal of garlic. Japan, just next door to Korea, has a diet similar to the Korean diet in all respects except one: It is fish-based instead of meat-based. In Japan, garlic is not regarded as an important part of the diet.

Many scientific studies over the last twenty years have shown that if rabbits, guinea pigs, and other animals are fed garlic together with cholesterol or butter in their diet, an increase in blood cholesterol levels is prevented completely. It is quite easy to demonstrate this with people as well. For example, in a study at the Cardiology Department of Rabindranath Tagore Medical College in India, a number of people were given a breakfast that included 3½ ounces of butter. This led to a 10-percent rise in blood cholesterol a few hours afterwards, and the blood also clotted more easily. However, when garlic juice or garlic oil was taken with the meal, these changes were completely prevented.

This can make us feel better about adding garlic to our butter and serving garlic toast at meals. However, this should not be taken as license for unrestrained feasting, relying on garlic as an antidote. That would be taking one step forward and two steps back, because it would not help the long-term program of reducing the amount of fat and cholesterol present in the bloodstream.

Q. How long should I take garlic? Will the benefits last even once I've discontinued?

A. Garlic will start to work as soon as you start to take it. However, your intake should continue for at least three months for more significant effects to occur. You can continue taking garlic at the right dosage as long as the cholesterol problem persists, but it would be best to make regular garlic consumption a permanent part of your diet. The reason for this is that once you stop taking garlic, the level of fat in the blood gradually returns to what it was before. If you want to keep your cholesterol low, you should make garlic one of your life habits.

Q. How does garlic work against cholesterol?

A. According to scientists, such as David Kritchevsky at the world-famous Wistar Institute in Philadelphia, garlic specifically slows down the whole "production line" that makes the cholesterol in the liver. In addition, studies conducted by the U.S. Department of Agriculture show that garlic helps the liver to remove the extra cholesterol in the form of bile, and then eliminate the bile from the body. This is also the way certain mild modern cholesterol-lowering drugs called fibrates work.

Q. How much garlic should I take daily to lower cholesterol and thin the blood?

A. You should take a minimum of one clove a day. Studies show that the more garlic you take, the greater the benefit, so two or even three cloves a day would be better, especially if the cholesterol problem is severe. However, there is no need to take huge doses of garlic all at once. In fact, it is advisable to split the dose, taking half in the morning and half in the evening.

3.

Garlic and Your Circulation

The effects of garlic on cholesterol are well-known and useful. But garlic helps the heart and the circulation in other ways too, such as by reducing blood clotting and blood pressure. In this chapter, you will learn about these additional benefits, and also how garlic fits in with the overall care of your heart and circulation. You will also learn that it is possible to actually reverse heart disease through a comprehensive health program that includes regular use of garlic.

Q. Has the benefit of garlic always been known, or is this a new discovery?

A. Garlic has always been known as a remedy to help the circulation. Traditional Indian medicine clearly states that garlic reduces fats, thins the blood, protects the heart, and strengthens the circulation.

Indeed, the ancient texts suggest that breast-feeding mothers should not take too much garlic because it might thin their milk. The European herbal tradition describes garlic as helpful in removing blood clots.

The recent interest in garlic and the heart apparently came from doctors on vacation in the sunny Mediterranean. They were surprised to find that the population of the Mediterranean countries consumed large quantities of meat, smoked many cigarettes, and guiltlessly enjoyed their coffee. Contrary to the doctors expectations and prior medical training, these people did not have an exceptionally high incidence of heart disease. In fact, they were tied with several other countries (such as Japan) in having the lowest incidence of heart disease in the world.

A thorough and careful analysis by researchers at the University of Western Ontario in Canada found that the more garlic a nation consumed, the less heart disease there was among its population. Scientists, however, were reluctant to give all the credit for this phenomenon to garlic. After all, it was possible that other factors, such as the heavy consumption of olive oil, salads, and rough country food, as well as a more easy-going lifestyle, could be contributing to the low incidence of heart disease in Mediterranean countries. While the people themselves insisted that the garlic was responsible for their good health, scientists weren't so sure. They felt they needed more conclusive statistics.

Q. Have scientists proven that garlic works?

A. Yes they have. To solve the problem, scientists compared three similar groups of people who differed in only one respect: the amount of garlic they consumed. In the 1970s, Dr. Sainani and his colleagues at the Sassoon General Hospital in Pune, India, found a pool of people from which to compose these groups: the Jains. Jains are members of a religious vegetarian Indian community, who all have similar diets except that some are accustomed to eating onion and garlic, while others traditionally abstain from them. Dr. Sainani assembled three groups. One group had a weekly consumption of at least 21 ounces of onion and 1.75 ounces of garlic (this comes to around seventeen cloves—a fairly substantial quantity). The second group took a weekly average of 7 ounces of onion and one-third ounce of garlic, and the third group ate no garlic or onion at all. It turned out that the amounts of cholesterol and fat in the blood of these individuals matched the garlic and onion consumption very closely. The heavy garlic eaters had 25-percent less cholesterol than the garlic avoiders. This would correspond to roughly a 50-percent decrease in heart attack risk.

Q. If I do have heart disease and atherosclerosis, will garlic reduce my symptoms?

A. Garlic can certainly help reduce the symptoms of heart disease. For example, Russian doctors have been using garlic preparations as a standard treatment for atherosclerosis, especially in the elderly. These doctors have reported improvement in many of their patients, symptoms, such as poor circulation in the legs and hands and tiredness. Recent studies of 300 patients in Zhenjiang, China, demonstrated that garlic brought about rapid improvement of symptoms such as headache, chest pain, tiredness, loss of appetite, and digestive problems. One relatively common and distressing problem that accompanies atherosclerosis is difficulty walking, due to an insufficient blood supply in the limbs. Garlic has been found to be very helpful in such cases. It enhances the effect of exercise, diet, and other treatments, although it works best before the problem has become very advanced.

A few caveats: Garlic will be most effective before your problem has become too severe. The sooner you start taking it, the easier it will be to prevent heart disease, or remedy an already existing problem. Keep in mind that garlic isn't a panacea. It works best in conjunction with other means, such as medication or remedies prescribed by your health professional, diet, and other self-care methods. And remember to keep taking it even once your symptoms have begun to resolve, because the problem may return if you discontinue the garlic.

Q. I have high blood pressure. Will garlic bring it down?

A. Garlic is an aid to reducing blood pressure. High blood pressure can be a result of any number of factors, including excessive salt intake, too much fluid in the body, imbalance in hormones, drinking too much coffee, the presence of toxins in the body, lack of exercise, poor flexibility of the vessels, atherosclerosis, and stress. In some of these cases, high blood pressure is quite easy to reverse with appropriate natural remedies, diet, and exercise. In other cases it is more difficult to reverse, and may require medication. High blood pressure increases the risk of heart problems, therefore you should take it very seriously. Seek proper professional advice to find the reason why you have high blood pressure, and then work to correct it.

The role of garlic here is as an adjunct to other remedies. It can bring down the blood pressure on its own, but only to a limited extent, and not in everyone. The effectiveness of garlic depends on the reason for the high blood pressure. Normal blood pressure is around 120 when the heart contracts, and 80 when the heart relaxes. Well-conducted medical investigations have found that a drop of between twelve and thirty points in the upper blood pressure, and seven to twenty points in the lower could be obtained by the regular administration of garlic to patients with elevated blood pressure. A small reduction often occurs in those with normal blood pressure.

In one study, researchers gave twenty patients tablets equivalent to about half a clove of garlic a day. These patients were compared to a similar group of patients who received reserpine, a standard drug. Within two weeks, the two measures of blood pressure in the garlic group dropped from 176 to 164, and 99 to 85, a decrease of about 10 percent overall. The effect of reserpine was more or less the same. In these studies, symptoms such as headache, dizziness, buzzing in the ears, and insomnia were considerably improved in the population taking garlic.

What is particularly significant is that, unlike conventional medications, garlic reduces both blood pressure and blood fat. Modern drugs used to treat blood pressure are rather specific and do not affect cholesterol. Medications designed to lower cholesterol do not necessarily have an impact on blood pressure. Garlic addresses both problems quite effectively.

Q. What are the benefits of thinning my blood?

A. The clotting process is a life-saving mechanism that seals cuts and stops the loss of blood. The process offers no danger as long as the blood flows easily and smoothly through the blood vessels within the body. However, if the vessels are narrowed and blocked by atherosclerosis, this life-saving mechanism operates against our interests. When blood clots block the vital coronary arteries, they precipitate a heart attack. When they block the blood vessels in the brain, they cause a stroke, and when they block the blood vessels in the leg, they cause venous thromboses and other dangerous problems. People with atherosclerosis are particularly at risk for all of these problems. They should work toward having blood that is not sticky or thick, and does not clot too easily. Reducing overall dietary fat, particularly saturated fats, and increasing the consumption of fish oils leads to thinner blood and more free-flowing circulation.

Q. Is garlic an effective blood-thinning remedy?

A. It's one of the best. Both garlic and onion are as effective as aspirin or other similar remedies, and considerably safer. Garlic also works immediately: Half an hour after taking it, the blood is noticeably thinner. Professor Boullin and colleagues at a British government hematology unit in Oxford, England, found that even small amounts of garlic could have noticeable effects on blood clotting. An hour after volunteers ate one-third of a clove, their blood took much longer to clot in the test tube, and the effect lasted for three to four hours This has been demonstrated in at least fifty studies, in animals as well as human beings. For example, in a study published in the journal *Atherosclerosis*, healthy people were given a very buttery breakfast and, as expected, it made their blood clot more easily. The usual clotting time is four minutes and fifteen seconds. After the high-cholesterol breakfast, it took only three minutes, forty-one seconds for their blood to clot. However, if garlic was added to the butter, it took five minutes, seven seconds to clot. This is even slower than normal.

Garlic does not only slow the clotting process. It increases the ability of the blood to break up already existing blood clots. Studies have shown that in heart patients, the clot-dissolving activity almost doubled during one month of garlic treatment. An analysis of fifteen clinical studies involving hundreds of subjects showed that garlic increased the clot-dispersing ability of the blood by an average of 60 percent. While the same result could be achieved after taking garlic for even one day, the effects tended to increase with time.

All these observations were so remarkable and well-defined, that the British medical journal *Lancet* once declared in an enthusiastic editorial that it had high hopes for a natural reduction in blood clotting by dietary factors, such as garlic or onion. However, onion cannot replace garlic as a disease preventive for the heart, because it does not have the other effects, such as lowering the levels of fats and cholesterol.

Q. Is it possible that some people should avoid garlic, because it will get in the way of healthy clotting?

A. You don't need to worry. The clotting tendency of people in developed countries is already too high because of the modern Western lifestyle and the fatty deposits in the blood vessels. Garlic simply brings the clotting to a more normal level. Moreover, there is no evidence that people who eat a very large amount of garlic in their daily diet have a problem with too much bleeding. In various studies, people have been given the equivalent of two heads of garlic a day (about twenty cloves) for months, without noticing any tendency to bleed excessively. However, please note that if garlic is being taken along with aspirin and anticoagulant drugs, the anti-clotting effects can be magnified. This will not normally be harmful, but it should perhaps be avoided in special situations in which clotting is essential, such as surgery.

Q. Will garlic alone prevent heart disease?

A. Garlic on its own will certainly help, especially if taken over a long period of time. However, it is unlikely that garlic will be sufficient to eliminate the risk of heart disease if your diet and lifestyle are potentially destructive. Garlic is most effective when used as part of an overall self-care regimen, especially a heart-healthy diet. It is not only the health of the arteries that will be improved. Common problems such as tiredness, headaches, obesity, colitis, arthritis, *Candida*, hypoglycemia, cancer, and lowered immunity can also be prevented in this way.

For example, garlic on its own will lower cholesterol by perhaps 10 to 15 percent. But garlic combined with a heart-healthy diet will lower cholesterol much more. This reinforcement was effectively demonstrated in a study by Professor E. Ernst of the University of Munich, published in the *British Medical Journal*. He studied two groups of patients who had high levels of cholesterol (above 260 mg per 100 ml). Both groups were given the same low-calorie diet. One group, however, also received garlic tablets equivalent to just under a clove of garlic a day. Those on the diet alone had 10-percent lower cholesterol at the end of the period. Those taking garlic as well achieved a further 10-percent reduction, adding up to 20 percent in all— enough to bring their cholesterol down to nearly normal levels. This study shows that garlic and diet work together for maximum results.

Q. Can clogged arteries and heart disease be reversed without medication or surgery?

A. They certainly can. I have seen it many times. This point of view is slowly becoming accepted by the medical community. Most doctors have erroneously assumed that once arteries are blocked, they can never become unblocked. They have believed that the only effective treatments for angina (chest pain) and high blood pressure are drugs or surgery. Now, with the publication of a landmark study by Dean Ornish, M.D., the medical world is more ready to believe that heart disease can be successfully treated without drugs or surgery. But it does need some dedication and persistence to make a real impact. A problem that has been accumulating invisibly for many years, in some cases since youth, cannot go away overnight. Garlic can stop things from getting worse, but it is not strong enough, on its own, to reverse blockages that have built up over many years. Blocked arteries can be opened completely by incorporating garlic into a broader health program, including other supplements and herbs, mild fasts, relaxation, radical reduction of fats, vegetarian diet, and aerobic exercise.

Q. Will garlic interfere with my medications? Can I use it as a substitute for medication?

A. Garlic will not interfere with any medication you are currently taking. But you should never stop taking your medication without consulting your health-care professional. Under competent professional guidance and supervision, you might be able to gradually discontinue your medication.

4.

Treating Those
Nagging Infections

Garlic is a powerful antibiotic. It has been described in Eastern Europe as "The Russian Penicillin," because a garlic product is widely sold in Russian pharmacies for use against all kinds of infections. It can kill all kinds of bacteria and fungi, and it's quite an effective way of dealing with many persistent infections, such as those of the teeth, throat, and chest. It is also the best natural medicine against *Candida* yeast infections. In this chapter you will discover how to use garlic as nature's antibiotic, when it should and should not be used, how it compares to conventional antibiotics, and the way to use it.

Q. Is garlic an effective remedy for colds and bronchitis?

A. Yes. Garlic is quite good at treating all kinds of infections in the body, including ear infections, teeth and gum infections, and chest and throat infections. This use of garlic has been known for a long time. Before the arrival of modern antibiotics, garlic was used as a natural antibiotic. For example in World War I and World War II, garlic was used by soldiers to treat infected wounds and also stomach infections. Even today, the health authorities in Great Britain allow manufacturers of garlic pills to print on their packages that garlic can be used for colds, catarrh, and chest problems. In folk traditions and in history, garlic was used primarily to treat these common diseases. Heart disease was much less of a focus than it is today. There are two reasons for this. The first is that the pre-modern lifestyle was less conducive to heart disease, and fewer people suffered from it. The second is that infections were harder to treat in the days before antibiotics. Infections were life-threatening in those days. Garlic must have saved many lives at a time when even a cut finger could be lethal.

Q. If I have a fever or a serious infection such as pneumonia, should I take garlic?

A. No. A serious infection must be combated quickly and powerfully with modern drugs such as antibiotics. Throughout history, garlic was used for serious infections such as tuberculosis because there was nothing else available in those days. Today we have modern drugs that work very quickly and effectively. Use them for serious infections. And don't use garlic if you have fever. There are many other helpful fever-reducing treatments.

Q. So what types of infections will garlic heal?

A. Garlic is appropriate for several different kinds of infection: infections that are mild and are not dangerous; infections that keep coming back, necessitating repeated doses of antibiotics; and nagging chronic infections. Examples include catarrh, bronchitis, cystitis, thrush, sore throat, skin infections such as athletes foot, sore throats, gum and teeth infections, stomach infections, and *Candida*. *Candida* is a yeast infection that has become a major problem today, causing a wide range of symptoms from allergies to depression. Interestingly, garlic has become the most important natural medicine that is used by thousands of holistic health professionals in the treatment of *Candida*.

Q. Is this use of garlic backed by scientific evidence?

A. Yes. Numerous studies conducted over many years support the use of garlic. Louis Pasteur, the famous bacteriologist, found to his surprise that the juice of garlic could kill bacteria growing in a laboratory dish. Since then, it has been shown again and again that garlic can kill a very wide range of bacteria and fungi that affect our health. Even a small amount of garlic can be effective. Garlic can kill bacteria that have become resistant to modern antibiotics. In one surprising study, Dr. Neil Caporaso and colleagues at New Jersey Medical University, fed large amounts of garlic to volunteers. They found that blood samples taken from these volunteers could kill nearby fungi in a laboratory culture dish. These scientists concluded that garlic could be a gentle alternative to antifungal drugs. Studies have shown that garlic can treat many kinds of animal diseases, such as skin infections. Scientists are still researching the success of garlic in treating infections in people.

Q. If garlic is so good at killing fungi, will it also act against parasites and worms?

A. Yes. It will work against worms, such as the threadworms that young children sometimes pick up. It is used in veterinary medicine to clear worms from animals. However, the modern drugs against worms are effective and safe, so these are usually preferred. Recently, Professor Mirelman, of the Weizmann Institute of Science in Israel, found that garlic could kill the amoebas that lead to amebic dysentery.

Q. How does garlic fight infection in the body?

A. Garlic fights infection by operating on two levels simultaneously. It kills the bacteria directly. However, it is now known that garlic also stimulates the proper function of the immune system. Studies have shown that garlic stimulates the cells of the immune system to go out and fight the bacteria that are invading. Certain types of infection-fighting white blood cells, called natural killer cells, become more active after exposure to garlic.

Q. If garlic can enhance our immunity, will it also work against viral infections?

A. Yes. There is some evidence that it will work against colds and viruses, not only against bacterial infections. For example, a small study of AIDS patients found that their white blood cells were better able to cope with viruses after three months of regular garlic supplements. Again, garlic is most effective in combination with other antiviral treatments, rather than by itself.

Q. Why should I take garlic if there are such good modern antibiotics available?

A. The main advantage of garlic over antibiotics is that garlic has far fewer side effects than antibiotics. Garlic can do no harm, even if it is taken over long periods of time. In addition, garlic builds the immune system, while antibiotics compromise the immune system.

As mentioned, garlic cannot substitute for antibiotics in the case of severe infection, because it is weaker than antibiotics and is about one-tenth as strong as the equivalent amount of penicillin. This is why it takes longer to work and is suitable only for milder infections. On the other hand, although garlic is slower-acting, it has a much wider range of action. Garlic deals with almost any kind of bacteria, while any given antibiotic only deals with a specific kind of bacteria. Garlic is a general remedy, while antibiotics are highly specialized. Sometimes several antibiotics must be tried before the appropriate one is found. Each round of antibiotics is a further assault on the immune system. For this reason, whenever possible, garlic should be used to treat mild infections, and antibiotics should be reserved only for serious infections.

Q. How do I take garlic to prevent infections?

A. It is the pungent compounds in garlic that work best against bacteria. The most potent compounds are formed right after the garlic is crushed. So if possible, use fresh garlic to treat infections. Crush the garlic, then add it to a hot lemon drink or clear soup to make it more palatable. Garlic products that

contain allicin are also effective, although not quite
as strong as fresh garlic.

5.

Detoxification and Cancer Prevention

Garlic is a strong cleansing or purifying herb that promotes the removal of toxins from the body. Its role in the prevention of cancer has received much media focus. It has been suggested that garlic can go beyond prevention and play a role in cancer treatment as well. In this chapter, we will explore how garlic removes toxins and helps our inner housecleaning. You will read the fascinating account of how garlic was discovered to have properties that fight cancer, and how you might use it to reduce your own risk of cancer.

Q. Is garlic used to treat cancer?

A. Yes and no. European and Russian folk medicine state that garlic in oil will reduce tumors and swellings. When scientists researched this claim, they found that in some cases garlic could slow down the growth of cancer cells. For example, a Howard University study found that large quantities of garlic injected into mice could slow the growth of their liver cancer by half. These studies, however, are not necessarily applicable to human beings. Moreover, there is a great difference between slowing the growth of a tumor and actually shrinking the tumor. For garlic to be an effective "treatment" of cancer, it would have to reduce and ultimately eliminate tumors, and there is no evidence at this time that garlic can accomplish such a formidable task. The present consensus among scientists and herbalists is that garlic is not strong enough to be an actual treatment for cancer. There are other herbs, such as Chinese herbs, which have stronger effects on the immunity and are more suitable for someone with cancer.

There are areas, however, in which garlic can be extremely useful as an adjunct to other forms of cancer treatment. Garlic, as we have seen, boosts the immune system. This can be helpful when the immunity is depressed as it is, for example, during chemotherapy. Garlic is most useful in the prevention of cancer, rather than in its treatment.

Q. How did scientists discover that garlic can help prevent cancer?

A. The old herbal lore, again, provided some clues. In Chinese medicine, for example, garlic is one of several items regarded as effective remedies to prevent cancer. Chinese scientists from Shandong Medical College researched this claim. They compared two populations in neighboring Chinese counties. Both populations—residents of Gangshan County and residents of Qixia County—led a similar lifestyle and ate an almost identical diet. There was only one significant difference in diet. People of Gangshan ate an average of six cloves of garlic a day, while in Qixia, no garlic was used. The scientists discovered that residents of Gangshan County had stomach cancer rates of 3.5 per 100,000, while residents of Qixia County, by contrast, had stomach cancer rates ten times higher!

The implications of this study have been replicated elsewhere as well. In fact, medical authorities all over are beginning to take garlic more seriously as a cancer preventive. For example, researchers at New York University carried out a major study confirming that garlic can protect the body from cells that are on their way to becoming cancerous. Several years ago, doctors in Iowa conducted a massive study of 40,000 women. The doctors explored the diet of these women, as well as cancer cases that appeared among them. Of all the foods, only garlic was clearly connected with a reduced risk of cancer.

Women who consumed one or more servings of garlic per week were, on average, 50-percent less likely to develop colon cancer. The general view today is that regular consumption of fruits and vegetables can help prevent cancer, and that garlic is one of the most important components of a cancer-preventive diet. This finding has been supported in nearly one hundred studies published to date. These suggest that there are several specific components of garlic that prevent cancer, and that actually stop cancer cells from changing and proliferating in the body.

Q. Do we know how garlic works as a cancer preventive?

A. Dr. Michael Wargovich at the University of Texas System Cancer Center has studied how this happens, and his work has received much media attention. He concluded that garlic helps the liver to break down cancer-causing chemicals. Garlic is rich in sulfur-containing compounds (hence the odor). These compounds are active in the liver. They help the body break down and remove the chemical toxins that can cause cancer. With this purer inner environment and some help to the immunity, the body is better able to prevent cancer. Sulfur compounds also keep normal cells from becoming cancerous.

Q. Can garlic's sulfur compounds help to detoxify the body from all kinds of unwanted chemicals?

A. Yes, very much so. The liver uses sulfur compounds as part of the natural housekeeping functions that sweep junk out of the body. These compounds get rid of all kinds of unwanted substances, such as food waste, chemical pollution, drugs, and even radiation. Garlic's sulfur compounds add power to those of the liver. Garlic is well known as a detoxifier. It makes us sweat, removing toxins from the skin. It removes them through the bile, and it chemically neutralizes them as well. Research has shown that garlic can remove from the body up to one-tenth of its weight of heavy metals such as lead or mercury. In one study, over 100 industrial workers took a garlic preparation daily, and it reduced the levels of lead and other contaminants in their blood.

We are living in a world contaminated by a large number of chemicals that our bodies are not equipped to deal with. Many of our modern diseases, including cancer, allergies, chronic fatigue, nervous diseases, dementias, and kidney disorders, may be caused by the load of toxins that the body has to carry. Garlic can help us to neutralize and remove many of these toxins. Garlic is particularly effective as part of a detoxification program. Combined with other supplements, exercise, saunas, and fasting, it can help in scrubbing out the wastes of modern life, making us feel better and healthier.

Q. Can garlic help with "hangovers"?

A. It probably can. The same mechanisms that are responsible for getting rid of other chemicals are responsible for getting rid of alcohol. According to the French, garlic is the best solution to a hangover. It is widely used in Europe for "the day after," and there is even a garlic and onion soup called "hangover soup" in France. "Garlic quickly dissipates drunkenness," reports a nineteenth century Frenchman. It may be a bit of a party stopper, but it will help get you on your feet again.

6.

Garlic, Past and Present

Throughout history, garlic has had both physical and symbolic significance in a variety of different cultures and civilizations. In this chapter, you will learn something about garlic's fascinating past history, and also the way holistic physicians and herbalists use it today. You will get an idea of the respect that has been given to this wonderful food and medicine since the beginnings of human civilization. You will learn where garlic comes from, the earliest references to it, what the great herbal experts of the ages have said about it, and how it is used in different cultures today.

Q. What is the earliest known use of garlic?

A. The earliest references to garlic are quite ancient indeed. Clay models of garlic were dug up in a tomb at El Mahasna in Egypt. They date back nearly 6,000 years. That is well before the time of the Pharaohs. The ancient Egyptians certainly valued the humble garlic. In fact, six perfectly dried garlic bulbs were found along with the gold and jewels in the tomb of the Pharaoh Tutankhamen. Inscriptions on the Great Pyramid give an account of the large amounts of garlic consumed by the builders. The Bible tells us that after the Jews left Egypt, they complained bitterly that they could no longer get their supply of garlic.

Q. Which civilizations used garlic for its many benefits?

A. The knowledge of garlic's many benefits was developed in North Africa, the Mediterranean civilizations, China, and India. Garlic was prized, for example, by the ancient Greeks. They valued it as a source of strength and also placed it at cross-roads as offerings to placate their gods. Garlic is even blamed for starting the Peloponnesian War, which led to the fall of Troy. According to the story, some young Greeks "primed with garlic" stole a princess, and so the war began and continued for thirty years.

The Romans saw garlic as a source of strength and even of aggression. Garlic was especially important to soldiers, who consumed large quantities to improve their stamina and military effectiveness. *Allia ne comedas* ("may you not eat garlic") was the Roman way of saying "may you not receive your call-up papers." The Romans were responsible for the spread of garlic to Northern Europe, because they planted garlic beneath the walls of their camps whenever they invaded a new territory. In India and China, too, garlic was very important. In ancient India, for example, garlic braids were hung all over villages during a special festival devoted to garlic. Most ancient people considered garlic so indispensable that they never traveled without it.

Q. I have heard that garlic was used to ward off evil spirits and vampires. Where did this belief come from?

A. Almost every civilization has some version of the notion that garlic wards off evil spirits or the evil eye. In ancient Greece and Egypt, for example, garlic was buried together with the corpse. The garlic was considered to be a gift to the gods of the lower worlds. In Eastern Europe, the legends surrounding garlic abound. The most common and famous legend concerns the notion that garlic can keep vampires at bay. The novel *Dracula* has made these beliefs famous. During the time of the Great Plague in Europe, the disease was assumed to arrive through some spirit, and garlic was always hung at the entrance to houses. Even today in Eastern Europe, garlic is put on a woman's pillow during childbirth, and in the child's clothes during baptism.

Here is one possible reason for the disproportionate role that garlic plays in magic and superstition. At a time when no one realized that infections are caused by bacteria and viruses, it was often assumed that diseases were passed on by evil spirits. Since garlic could prevent and cure infections, it was seen as chasing away these spirits. But there is another perhaps more interesting reason for the supersticious beliefs behind garlic. One Islamic legend suggests that when Satan was thrown out of Paradise, garlic grew on any land touched by his foot. This fanciful tale points to the apparent paradox of garlic. On the one hand, garlic contains almost heavenly properties. It purifies, cleanses, and detoxifies the body. It cures diseases and adds flavor to foods. On the other hand, there is something hellish about it too. The odor can be unpleasant, and the flavor can be overwhelming. This may be another reason for all the beliefs and legends about it.

Q. What did the early civilizations use garlic for?

A. Most ancient peoples certainly used garlic as a food. Records from the Egyptian, Greek, and Roman periods give numerous recipes for garlic dishes. It seems to have been added to just about everything. As a medicine, it also had an extraordinarily wide use. Lists of garlic recipes appeared in the earliest medical records that we know of—the medical manuscripts of ancient Egypt. Hippocrates, the Greek father of medicine, wrote that for infections a man should eat a lot of raw garlic and drink pure wine, then go to bed. The famous Greek physician Dioscorides provided an extensive list of the medical benefits of garlic. He wrote that because garlic is sharp and pungent, it stimulates thirst, thereby increasing urination and helping in the elimination of tapeworm. According to Dioscorides, garlic makes the voice clear and soothes continuous coughing. It kills lice and clears the arteries. He also recommended that garlic be used in combination with other items. Together with salt and oil, garlic heals skin problems; with honey, it heals boils and other skin eruptions. Boiled with pine-wood and incense, it heals toothaches.

Other Greek and Roman authorities added to the

list all of the medical problems that might be successfully addressed through the use of garlic. The list includes tumors, parasites such as those that cause malaria, and ear infections. Garlic was seen as an energy-producing food and was regarded as a general tonic. Folk practitioners all over the world have always used it. For example, traditional midwives in the Middle East give a great deal of garlic to women for ten days after childbirth to prevent infections and build strength. Gypsies are famous users of garlic. One of their classic medicines for a cough is fresh garlic boiled in milk. Russian folk medicine suggests garlic and onion mixed with honey or vinegar as a general health tonic, especially for the elderly. There are also uses that strike us, with our modern sensitivities, as peculiar. Most folk traditions regard garlic as an aphrodisiac, but today we might regard it as the opposite because of its smell.

Q. How would a modern-day herbalist or holistic physician use garlic?

A. Today's health practitioners use garlic to address an array of physical problems, most of which have been covered in this book. For example, it was herbalists that showed the scientists that garlic thins the blood. Holistic physicians in India, practicing the

Indian system of medicine, have always administered garlic to people with too much fat in their bloodstreams. In China, people use it a great deal for worms, parasites, and stomach infections. The Oriental medical doctors also prescribe garlic plasters for boils and garlic in combination with other herbs for all kinds of infections, including coughs and tuberculosis. Dr. Albert Schweizer, one of the most famous physicians of modern times, used garlic against cholera and typhoid at his mission hospital in Africa. Modern herbalists prescribe garlic products for almost all circulatory problems and fresh extracts for bronchial infections, tonsillitis, abscesses, *Candida*, and other infections.

7.

Potency, Preparations, and Products

In this chapter we cover all of your important questions regarding the actual use of garlic. We dissect the garlic bulb and examine what particular components of it contain medicinal benefits. We discuss how to take garlic, how much to take, and what you can do about the pungent smell and powerful taste. We will provide guidelines so that you know what to look for and how to distinguish between different kinds of garlic products.

Q. What exactly is in garlic that makes it work so well?

A. As we have discussed elsewhere in this book, the key to garlic's potency is found in one element: sulfur.

It took scientists a great deal of time to isolate and identify sulfur as the main secret of garlic's strength.

A whole clove of garlic contains a large amount of a very unusual sulfur compound called alliin. This alliin contains neither odor nor taste. You may have noticed that a whole clove doesn't actually smell. The bombshell of smell and taste bursts only when garlic is crushed or chopped. When that happens, the alliin is transformed into a new compound, allicin, which has a strong, burning taste and a strong smell. This allicin is the basic potent substance of garlic. It is responsible for many of garlic's health-giving properties. Once it's been formed, it changes into a whole family of other sulfur compounds, called sulfides, which are part of the healthy cocktail within the garlic plant.

Q. Does that mean that garlic doesn't work as a medicine unless it is crushed or chopped?

A. Exactly. A whole or even cut garlic clove will not be medicinally helpful. The same is true if we cook garlic before chopping it, for in that case the transformation from alliin to allicin is prevented by the cooking. Unless allicin or its daughter compounds are present, garlic will not be effective.

Q. So what can I do about the odor?

A. Most garlic breath comes from chewing garlic in the mouth, so the best way to avoid the problem is by eating it without chewing it. Fresh garlic can be crushed into milk, warm soup, or as the gypsies recommend, into yogurt, and then swallowed with one gulp. There are foods that will neutralize the odor. Eating some parsley or lettuce after your garlic can remove much of the odor. You can also chew a few seeds of fennel or aniseed, or drink mint tea. You can find some creative ways to make garlic suit your habits. One day, a visitor to my house was amazed to see my daughter, who was then six years old, cutting cloves of garlic into long slices. Then, with great concentration, she inserted them into grapes. "What on earth are you doing?" he asked. "Preparing my medicine," she answered, and popped one into her mouth.

These methods will prevent the odor of garlic from affecting the mouth, but there is still some odor that emerges from the stomach and digestion. The only way that this smell can be drastically reduced is by taking garlic products and supplements rather than fresh garlic. For many of us, this is a very convenient way of healing the heart and dealing with the nose at the same time.

Q. Are garlic products and supplements as effective as fresh garlic?

A. They are not quite as effective, but they come very close. It depends on which products you are taking and your reason for taking them. In general, fresh garlic is much better than garlic products for infections, because the high level of the pungent allicin in freshly crushed garlic is very unwelcome to the bacteria and fungi. Fresh garlic is also better for cleaning the body and inducing sweating. However, for the all-important effects on cholesterol and the circulation, and as a general preventive against cancer and other diseases, garlic products are nearly as good as fresh garlic.

Q. There are so many different products in the stores. Which ones are best?

A. There are several types of products. They can be grouped into three categories.

The first is the dried garlic tablet. This is probably the best garlic product available on the market. These tablets are made by slicing garlic and then drying the slices in a specific way to preserve their potency. They contain most of the alliin, the original active compound. When they dissolve in the stomach, this alliin is converted to allicin, just as it is when fresh garlic is crushed. The good news is that the malodorous allicin is released way down in the digestive system, so there is very little odor from the mouth. For this reason, these dried garlic tablets are often called "odor controlled." It is advisable to buy "guaranteed potency" products that tell you specifically how much allicin they release. Garlic tablets have been subjected to many clinical trials, and they achieve the same results as fresh garlic.

Capsules containing garlic oil are second best. These are made by extracting the oily sulfur compounds from garlic and mixing them with vegetable oil. It is a traditional method of preparing garlic products, and it has been widely used in Europe for many years. The capsules containing garlic oil have a generally good informal reputation for their effectiveness, but they have not performed so well in clinical studies. There is sometimes too little garlic oil in them, and the potency cannot be guaranteed.

The third and least effective item is deodorized garlic, which comes in capsule or tablet form. This product is made by allowing garlic pieces to age in alcohol for a long time, and then making an extract that is put into capsules or tablets. The process prevents the formation of allicin and the strong-smelling sulfides. The advantage, of course, is that the product does not smell at all. The disadvantage, however, is that the absence of allicin means that the product is considerably less effective. This type of supplement has not been proven in clinical trials on lowering cholesterol, so it may not be appropriate for helping the heart. There is, however, some evidence to suggest that it can, nonetheless, be helpful as a cancer preventive and an agent of detoxification.

Q. Each garlic product seems to have a different recommended dosage. How much supplement am I supposed to take?

A. You are right. Each manufacturer uses a different dose in preparation of the product; and besides, different ways of preparing garlic lead to different concentrations of constituents. This creates great confusion for the consumer. It would be wonderful if all the manufacturers could express their dosages as: "equivalent to such-and-such number of grams of fresh garlic."

The correct dose of fresh garlic is between one and two cloves of garlic a day for cardiac health, and more for treating infections. This is a minimum of a little over one-tenth of an ounce of fresh garlic per day. What is the correct dose of dried garlic tablets? Since fresh garlic is about two-thirds water, you will need to take a daily dose of at least 1 gram of tablets of dried garlic; for example, two tablets of 500 mg daily. The correct dose of concentrated extract or garlic oil varies depending on the different brands. Each package should clearly state how much correspondence there is between the enclosed tablet and the equivalent amount of fresh garlic. You should calculate how much to take to reach the daily minimum equivalent to a little over one-tenth of an ounce each day.

Q. Can garlic be prepared in other forms for medicinal purposes?

A. There are hundreds of ways to prepare garlic. You can experiment to find your own form. Here are some classics:

You can make garlic syrup. This method creates a long-lasting medicine for coughs, colds, bronchitis, and similar problems. It seems to keep its power remarkably well. Put about a half pound of crushed garlic in a one-quart jar. Fill the jar almost to the top with cider vinegar and water, cover, and leave for a few days, shaking occasionally. Strain through a cloth. Then add 1 cup of honey, stir, and keep in the refrigerator. One tablespoon, three times a day, will give the correct dose.

You can also add garlic to miso soup. Miso, or

Japanese soybean extract, makes an excellent hot soup, ideal to take with garlic. Dissolve a teaspoonful of miso in just-boiled water. Add a couple drips of soy sauce, a good squeeze of lemon, some grated onion, and a crushed clove or two of garlic. This is especially good for convalescence and recovery, bringing strength as well as healing.

Garlic can be mixed into oil. Crush 8 ounces of garlic into a jar. Add enough virgin olive oil to cover the garlic. Allow it to stand in a warm place for three days, and strain. Add a few drops of essential oil, such as eucalyptus or cypress. Use a few drops of the garlic oil for earaches, and rub it on the chest for coughs. This oil preparation is also useful for the circulation.

Fresh garlic can be rubbed directly onto the skin. If your skin is not excessively sensitive, you can simply crush garlic onto a small piece of lint, place it on the area, and tape it. There may be some burning sensation, which passes in a few minutes. If the burning becomes too intense, especially in a sensitive area such as the gums, you can reduce the potency by using garlic that has been left standing for thirty minutes after crushing. Crushed fresh garlic is particularly helpful for athlete's foot, fungal infections, stings, *Candida* in the urogenital area, or tooth and gum infections.

Q. Can you give me a few cooking tips on how I can use garlic in different dishes?

A. The most important tip to using garlic in a healthful fashion is to crush it before use. If you are cooking with garlic, add it close to the end of the cooking process. There is a staggering range of dishes that can be improved by garlic, both in terms of health and in terms of flavor. Here are a few, just to open up some new avenues of culinary thought for you.

Garlic tips for vegetable dishes: Garlic goes well with almost any soup, including vegetable and chicken broths. It can be crushed and added in mid-cooking to enrich the taste of pies and quiches, as well as stews and casseroles. It goes well with potatoes and other root vegetables. Garlic is wonderful in pickles, sauces, mushroom dishes, and salad dressings. For example, virgin olive oil, together with lemon, cider vinegar, garlic, and small quantities of mustard and herbs, is the best basic salad dressing. Garlic goes well with lemon or soy sauce on avocados, which are rich in natural oils.

Garlic tips for carbohydrate dishes: Garlic can be added to dips and spreads for use with whole-grain bread or crackers. A classic Middle Eastern dip that is excellent for the circulation consists of olive oil, squeezed lemon, garlic, and marjoram mixed together. Use it in pasta sauces, and add it to fried dishes such as risottos, or to rice dishes. Add fresh garlic to a little olive oil and spread on fresh whole-grain bread before warming it in the oven. It tastes quite similar to garlic butter.

Garlic tips for protein dishes: Garlic goes well with lean meat, especially in French garlic sauces. Garlic also goes well with fish, especially with parsley. You can add crushed garlic and dill to curd cheese to give it a rich, aromatic flavor. Crushed garlic is a necessary addition to hummus (chick pea paste) and tahini (Greek and Middle Eastern ground sesame) and cooked soy beans. Add a little garlic and yeast extract to nut roasts, lentils, and bean dishes.

Garlic tips for fats and oils: Garlic is fried in oil, often with onion, in Indian and Chinese cooking and in other ethnic dishes. The oil is then used as the basis for numerous dishes, such as curries.

Conclusion

You have learned a good deal about garlic. Now it is time to put this book down, go out, and try it for yourself. If you have never tried natural remedies before, the concept of self-treatment and natural approaches might be new and foreign to you. Remember that before the advent of modern medicine (only about 100 years ago!) people treated their illnesses, both major and minor, with an array of natural remedies, such as garlic. Modern medicine has made valuable and even life-saving contributions to the world but, sadly, has led to a situation in which people have forgotten the vast ancient knowledge of God-given health aids. Many of these healing agents can be as effective as many modern medicines—and ever so much safer. So whether your first port of call is the kitchen or the health foods store, be aware that you are following a long and wise tradition. Throughout history, individuals such as yourself have been using natural remedies to maximize their health and prevent disease. So there is nothing strange about it. Indeed, remembering this ancient treasure trove of knowledge can only enhance our health today.

Once you begin to work with garlic and other remedies, a whole new area of self-care will begin to open up. You will begin to feel the wonderful sense of being in charge of your own health and making your own independent choices. As you educate yourself further (start with the Suggested Readings list that follows), you will acquaint yourself with the vast array of natural remedies available to you, and their myriad uses. You can then begin to incorporate these remedies into your daily lifestyle. Because there are so many herbs, spices, and supplements available, you might feel overwhelmed and confused at the beginning. My advice is to start slowly. Begin by taking one dietary supplement, such as garlic. Then increase to two, then three, and so on. Start with mild herbs, such as ginger, chamomile, and echinacea, for non-serious health problems. See what they can do for you, and then begin to expand your repertoire.

This is how I began my own involvement with herbs more than twenty years ago. The results have been extraordinary. My family and I have not needed any conventional drugs since then. If one of us gets sick, I go into the garden or the kitchen and prepare the natural remedies that are necessary.

This was not an overnight process for me, and it won't be for you either, so don't expect instant results. You have to give the supplements and herbs time to work and make sure that you take a sufficient dosage.

But will they work? The answer is an unequivocal yes. Medicinal herbs can work miracles. It is up to us to give them a chance.

Glossary

Alliums. The group of plants similar to garlic, such as onion, chives, leek, and ransoms (wild garlic).

Atherosclerosis. A lifelong process in which blood vessels are gradually blocked by deposits of fat and cholesterol.

Candida. A kind of yeast that can live in the blood and tissues, causing a variety of symptoms, such as allergies and depression.

Cholesterol. The fatty material made by the liver and present in some foods that becomes deposited in the blood vessels, causing heart disease.

Clotting. The natural process in which blood congeals so as to seal up cuts and wounds.

High blood pressure (Hypertension). A situation in which the heart has to pump harder to keep the blood flowing, primarily because of narrowing of the blood vessels and because of tension.

Thrombosis. A clot within the blood vessels that can block them, causing strokes or heart attacks.

Toxins. Chemicals, pesticides, and other unwanted substances that accumulate in our bodies and gradualiy damage our health.

References

Belman S, "Onion and garlic oils and tumour promotion," *Carcinogenesis* 4 (1983): 1063–1065.

Block E, "The chemistry of garlic and onions," *Scientific American* 252 (1985): 94–97.

Bordia A, Verma SK, "Effect of garlic feeding on regression of experimental atherosclerosis in rabbits," *Artery* 7 (1980): 428–437.

Bordia A, "Effect of garlic on blood lipids in patients with coronary heart disease," *American Journal of Clinical Nutrition* 34 (1981): 200–203.

Boullin DJ, "Garlic as a platelet inhibitor," *Lancet* 1 (1981): 776–777.

Caporaso L, et al., "Antifungal activity in human urine and serum after ingestion of garlic *(Allium sativum),*" *Antimicrobiol Agents Chemotherapy* 23 (1983): 700–702.

Chi MS, et al., "Effects of garlic on lipid metabolism in rats fed cholesterol or lard," *Journal of Nutrition* 112 (1982): 41–48.

De A Santos OS, Grunwald, J, "Effect of garlic powder tablets on blood lipids and blood pressure: a six month, placebo controlled, double-blind study," *British Journal of Clinical Research* 4 (1993): 37–44.

Dorant E, et al., "Garlic and its significance in the prevention of cancer in humans, a critical review," *British Journal of Cancer* 67 (1993): 424–429.

Ernst E, et al., "Garlic and blood lipids," *British Medical Journal* 291 (1985): 139.

Fenwick GR, Hanley AB, "The genus allium," Parts 1–3, *Critical Reviews on Food Science*, Vols 22 and 23 (1986).

Foushee DB, et al., "Garlic as a natural agent for the treatment of hypertension: a preliminary report," *Cytobios* 34 (1982): 145–152.

Hughes BG, Lawson LD, "Antimicrobial effects of *Allium sativum L.* (garlic), *Allium ampeloprasum* (elephant garlic), and *Allium cepa* (onion), garlic compounds and commercial garlic supplement products," *Phytotherapy Research* 5 (1991): 154–158.

Jain AK, Vargas R, Gotzkowsky S, MacMahon FG, "Can garlic reduce levels of serum lipids? A controlled clinical study," *American Journal of Medicine* 94 (1993): 632–635.

Keyes A, "Wine, garlic and CHD in seven countries," *Lancet* (1980): 145–146.

Lawson LD, "Bioactive organosulfur compounds of garlic and garlic products: role in reducing blood lipids," in *Human Medicinal Agents from Plants*, ed. Kinghorn AD, Balandrin MF (Washington, DC: American Chemical Society Books, 1993).

Mader FH, "Treatment of hyperlipidaemia with garlic-powder tablets," *Drug Research* 40 (1990): 1111–1116.

Moore GS, Atkins RD, "Fungicidal and fungistatic effects of an aqueous garlic extract on medically important yeast-like fungi," *Mycologia* 69 (1997): 341–348.

Sainani BS, et al., "Effect of dietary garlic and onion on serum lipid profile in a Jain community," *Indian Journal of Medical Research* 69 (1979): 776–780.

Silagy C, Neil A, "Garlic as a lipid-lowering agent: a meta-analysis," *Journal of the Royal College of Physicians* 28 (1994): 39–45.

Steinmetz KA, et al., "Vegetables, fruit and colon cancer in the Iowa Women's Health Study," *American Journal of Epidemiology* 139: 1–15.

Wargovich MJ, "Inhibition of gastrointestinal cancer by organosulfur compounds in garlic," *Cancer Chemoprevention* (1992): 195–203.

Suggested Readings

Baker S and Sbraga M. *The Unabashed Garlic & Onion Lover's International Cookbook*. Garden City Park, NY: Avery Publishing Group, 1997.

Fulder S. *The Garlic Book*. Garden City Park, NY: Avery Publishing Group, 1997.

Heber D. *Natural Remedies for a Healthy Heart*. Garden City Park, NY: Avery Publishing Group, 1998.

Koch HP and Lawson LD. *Garlic—The Science and Therapeutic Application of Allium sativum L. and Related Species*. Baltimore, MD: Williams and Wilkins, 1996.

Ody P. *The Complete Medicinal Herbal*. London, New York: Dorling Kindersley, 1993.

Tyler VE. *Herbs of Choice*. Binghamton, NY: Pharmaceutical Products Press, Haworth Press, 1993.

Index